#HardWorkPaysOff

How to "MEAL PREP" like a
Fitness Pro

Diary of a Fit Mommy

———————

Author: Danielle Richardson

#HardWork Pays Off

Copyright © 2015 by Danielle Richardson

ISBN 13: 978-1511553407
ISBN 10: 1511553405

Printed in USA by Amazon.com/Creatspace
Publisher: JMC Publishing
Chief Editor: Vivian S. Matthews
Graphics Design: Ashley Photographik Cleveland

Table of Contents

Preface

This book was written to make conquering a healthy lifestyle and choices we make a little easier. We live in a world in which time is of the essence and very limited. So this book gives you a quick fix on how to prepare meals and gives you a peek into my healthy lifestyle of fitness and clean eating. I tend to share my struggles of getting to the point where meal prep has become a healthy habit and how I am benefiting from it on a daily basis. It takes planning to plan successfully.

Introduction

The purpose of this book is to educate people on the importance of meal preparation, how you can save time and make healthy choices that can ultimately save your life. My goal is to get you to understand that eating healthy doesn't have to be a burden on your pockets or your time. I want you to keep in mind that you should eat to live not live to eat! I will also provide you with easy yet tasteful meals that will make your goal of weight loss or maintenance a success. Remember, I am not a fitness guru or instructor, nor did I take any classes on how to meal prep. I am someone who made up her mind to make this journey easier! I'm a real person getting real results. It is a journey and I am here to help every step of the way!

"Deciding"

The one thing we have full control over is our choices or decisions. Before you can do anything and do it successfully you have to decide. You have to decide to do it, why you should do it, when to do it and how to do it.

My biggest obstacle with weight loss or maintenance was what to eat. For me, deciding to work out was easy but choosing the right foods and having time to prepare it became a burden. Along with what to cook or eat, knowing how much to eat was another issue. After learning through trial and error, I realized that I was making it much more complicated for myself.

When it comes to obtaining and maintaining a healthy lifestyle, it is as easy or as complicated as you make it. You should know that everything doesn't work for everybody. You have to know your body and what your daily activity level and originate a plan that works for you. However, meal preparation is key and I intend to show you how to simplify your life.

You must decide what your goals are and work towards those goals. A life of fitness is a process. People are confused about the word "fitness". Overall, fitness means good health. It does not mean you have to become a body builder, have a body like someone else, but it does mean you need to become the best "you" possible. This is accomplished by proper nutrition and exercise. It is a battle at times and if someone tells you it isn't, RUN! However, when you are equipped for the battle you will come out victorious! I am not telling you something I heard to be true but my real life experiences.

The first battle you need to conquer is the battle of the mind. Once you make up your mind there is no stopping you. When doing something repeatedly over a period of time it becomes a habit and living a healthy life is a good one. I feel society has made it too easy for us to live unhealthy lives. There are so many fast food restaurants and drive thru windows that are literally driving us to our graves. The companies take advantage of our lack of time. According to Statist, Inc. (2015), in the U.S. there are approximately 119.3 million people who work full-time (35+ hours per week). So time is very limited for us all. These companies know we are living in a time where people have no time. It is easier to eat fast food then it is to cook a meal and not to mention the companies have made fast food more affordable. My ultimate goal is to get you to eat healthier, stay within a budget and make better decisions.

As I previously stated, I am not someone who studied how to lose weight, took classes or certified trainer (yet). I am simply someone who decided to take control of her life. This decision wasn't easy and when I visited a few gyms, they would give me a long menu, which by the way was great but looked overwhelming. It not only looked overwhelming but also seemed expensive. So I struggled with it and decided I would workout and eat whatever I wanted. Wrong decision because I totally feel when living a healthy life it is the 80/20 rule. Eighty percent nutrition and twenty percent exercise. You need both to reach your goals.

Another huge mistake I would make was not eating or not eating enough. After I got past the eating whatever I wanted stage, I thought well if I skipped some meals I would balance out my caloric intake. I was on a road of complete destruction. I damaged my metabolism, I believe it shut down because I was never hungry and still wasn't reaching my goals physically. You have to eat to lose and to maintain. I learned the hard way.

"You're Worth It"

The only person who has control over your decisions is you! It's your choice how you choose to live your life. Often we put others before ourselves but now it's time to do something for you. Make the choice to live a healthy, balanced and fulfilling life.

You have to know your worth! The time it takes to prepare for the things of tomorrow is minimal compared to spending a lifetime with regrets. Living with that "what if" hanging over your head is not healthy mentally. Do what you need to do to become the best you.

Meal prepping is nothing more than preparing food in bulk and sorting it out into portions. You are worth the time and effort. Instead of taking 1-2 hours preparing one meal, make a sufficient amount to last throughout the week. It's just that simple! It looks more complicated than it really is and anyone can do it. I haven't invented anything new. However, I've decided to give meal prepping the attention it deserves. While my Meal Prep Service is in the works, I decided to give you a chance to experience it for yourself. The benefits from it are awesome and so worth the time. When you start seeing the results, then you too will appreciate it.

"The Struggle"

Fitness is new to me but losing and gaining weight isn't. Let me explain. I found myself gaining weight after I had my daughter almost 19 years ago. However, I managed to lose and gain it back over and over again. I felt with the advantage of being young I could eat whatever I wanted when I wanted to. I have to laugh at that now. Again, my mentality was if I looked skinny or thin then I was healthy. This is farthest from the truth! Six years after I had my daughter, I gave birth to my son. When he was 3 years old I had to have a hysterectomy and at that time I was 28 years old. My metabolism has not been the same since having the surgery. It was and still is a struggle. People may not know your situation, that's why it is so important for you to know your body. I was doing everything my trainer at the time was telling me to do but it was not working for me. They had no idea what I was going through and made me feel like I was a failure. By the way, there are things you can do to speed up your metabolism. For me it was eat more and eat more frequently. I had to eat 6 healthy meals (3 meals 3 snacks) daily. I learned this from a weight-loss program I enrolled in. It was successful but expensive.

So let's talk a little about this weight-loss program. Yes, it was successful and I managed to drop over 40 lbs., however, I never exercised. I was not encouraged to do so it was all about eating and buying their products. In doing so, I lost more than my goal weight. I have to say I looked good according to my standards because I was aiming for skinny and not healthy/fit. I did not realize my lack of energy was a sign that something wasn't quite right. I also didn't realize how skinny I looked until someone brought it to my attention. I lost so much weight too fast. When that happens that is a setup for failure and possible health issues. You have to have both nutrition and exercise in mind when trying to acquire a healthy lifestyle.

Needless to say I gained the weight back and I was miserable. I started with my old eating habits and less activity. While participating in this weight-loss program I only gained half of what it takes to obtain and maintain a healthy lifestyle. I had the nutrition, but my way of thinking wasn't in the right place. Remember the true meaning of fitness. Know that you need people in your life that are going to support you and help you accomplish your goals.

In order to accomplish your goals you need to come up with a P.O.A. (plan of action). Notice I didn't say a plan but a plan of action. You can have a plan, but no plan on how to execute it. You need to establish realistic goals. For example if you are a size 14, don't set a goal of becoming a size 8 in 30-60 days. If you are trying to lose weight, do not become a "scale hopper". A scale hopper gets on the scale every chance they get just to see if they have lost weight. You begin to become obsessed with the number. It should never be about the number! I go by the fit of my clothing and how I feel. If I feel or see progress then that is what's important and matters most to me. That means I am losing inches and fat is going "bye-bye". (LOL) I used to jump on the scale repeatedly throughout the day because with the weight loss program we had to monitor and log our weight. I became obsessed and would literally get upset if there were no changes. The mind is powerful and with discouragement it can cause you to say forget it all. Then you are back to square one. So again, set realistic goals and remember you have to eat, choose wisely and skipping meals should not be an option.

"The Big Change"

There are times when emotions get the best of us. For some people, food can become an outlet or find comfort in it. I remember this time last year I was going through something that was really overwhelming. I didn't at the time realize how much I was over indulging until one day I couldn't fit my clothes. I was so disgusted. I am just being honest. I started going to the gym and I thought I was making the proper food choices but knowing what I know now, it was far from it. I wasn't making the progress I expected even with my crazy workout sessions. I needed to make a huge adjustment and so I did.

I made the "big change". I totally changed the way I consumed food and switched up my workout routines. I eat 6 times a day and workout 5/6 times a week. I added Boot Camps to my routine and high intensity weight training. One thing I changed as far as eating is MEAL PREPPING and that's what this book is all about. I wanted to first share with you some of my experiences and to keep it real with you. I struggled prior to realizing that change was necessary in order to define my lifestyle as healthy. I will show and explain to you step by step how I meal prep. It is cost effective and so worth it. Meal prepping keeps you from making bad food choices and having these prepped meals at your fingertips makes life so much easier.

"Meal Prep"

Our society today is always on the go. Some leave early in the morning and may not return until late at night. During this time it is easy to eat whatever is available to you. This hinders you from eating as healthy as you would like to. This is why Meal Preparation is so important. It makes eating the right foods more convenient and available immediately. It also saves us time. It may seem like a lot to do all at once but I will show you how and save money doing it.

The Start Up

List of items you will need to get started:

- Plenty of storage containers
- Your choice of lean protein (chicken breast, fish: tilapia, cod, salmon, albacore tuna, etc.)
- If you are vegan stock up on legumes, quinoa, nuts, etc.
- Variety of veggies (can buy a weeks worth)
- Seasonings without SALT (example: Italian season blend, pepper, garlic powder, onion powder, Mrs. Dash, etc.), sea salt is an option
- Fruits of your choice

As meal prepping becomes routine, you will know what you need and how much. Do not try to over d0 it or over extend yourself, it will get easier and keep it simple.

Meal planning: Easy as 1-2-3...

Choose from each food group

1. Lean Protein
2. Vegetable
3. Healthy Fat
4. Carbohydrate (optional): whole grain product or low starch vegetable

Protein Prep

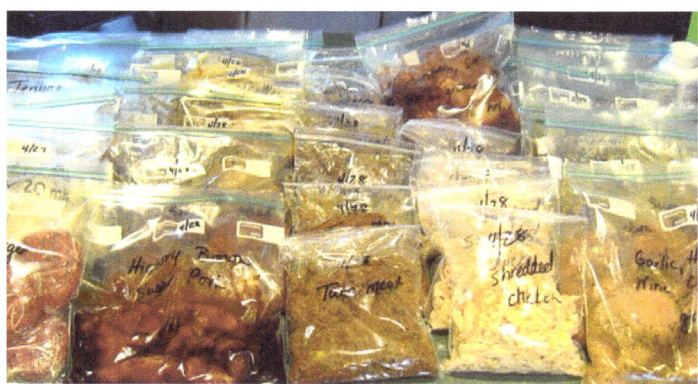

When prepping lean protein, which consists of chicken, turkey and fish, I buy them in bulk. It saves you money. Freezing portions of it will also save you money. If you continuously buy small packs you will end up spending more money in the long run. We want our finances healthy as well!

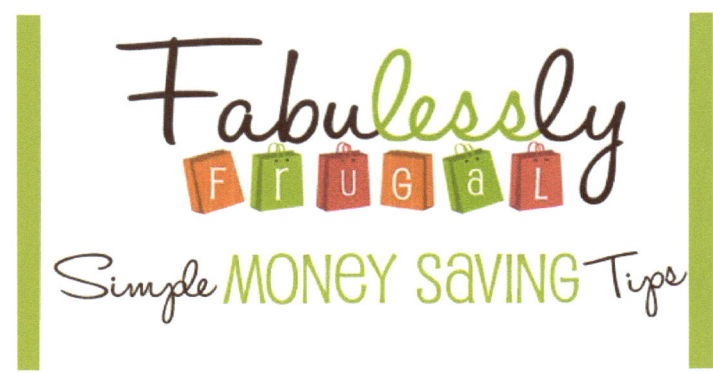

MONEY SAVING TIPS:

I suggest buying thick cut chicken breast. I can usually get 3-4 slices from one chicken breast! TRY IT! So if there are six chicken breasts in a pack and can get 4 slices out each that gives me 24 pieces. You can choose to cook them all and freeze them in portions. If you choose not to cook all the chicken breasts you can still pack what you don't use in freezer bags and store them for later use.

Buy your produce at Farmer's Markets. They are cheaper by the pound and have more of a variety of options. I store a lot of fruits & veggies in the refrigerator. They tend to last for a longer period of time. The longer they last the more money you save.

Plan your menu for the week so you won't over spend. Make a list of ingredients and stick to it. Use coupons as often as possible. It's amazing how much things cost when maintaining a healthy lifestyle. It's almost as if companies want our eating habits to be unhealthy.

TIME SAVING TIP: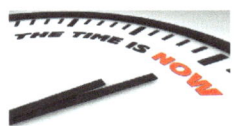

You can cook all of the chicken breast then slice them up and put them in individual freezer bags. When it is time to use the strips, you can pop them in the oven and put them in a salad for lunch or dinner.

The same goes for your vegetables. You can prepare those in advance as well. For example, when preparing my veggies you do not have to cook them all at once. To save time, you can cut them up and place them in freezer bags or containers as well. It is strictly up to you how you prepare your meals. There are some you may only want to prepare a few days at a time. I work full-time so I choose to prepare for the entire week, Monday-Friday. If I over sleep or running late, foods not something I have to worry about. I just grab and go! Once you start meal prepping you will see just how easy it is and how much time you have to accomplish other tasks.

I have done some research and found most people make poor food choices due to lack of time. They want homemade meals but no time to make them. Fast food is just that fast with little to no nutritional value. Here is the solution. It takes work but the reward is great! #HARDWORK Pays Off!

Sample Menus

I have heard from many that they just do not know what to cook. So I am providing you with a few ideas for meal prepping for either lunch or dinner. I will also give you a peek into what a week of meal prep looks like for me.

Sample for weekly Meal Prep

<u>Monday</u>
Grilled chicken breast (strips or whole)
Asparagus (sautéed in olive oil & fresh garlic)
Mulit-color peppers (sautéed in olive oil)
Brown rice (cook with chicken broth for flavor)

<u>Tuesday</u>
Baked Tilapia
Mashed yams (or whole yam)
Broccoli

Wednesday
Grilled chicken on 100% whole-wheat pita with tomato, lettuce & a little mozzarella cheese
Garden salad

Thursday
Baked Tilapia
Mixed veggies
Quinoa

Friday
Baked Salmon
Cauliflower
Salad

Remember, it is important to have protein, good carb & vegetable for every meal. You may need to adjust your intake according to your specific goals. These were a few examples of a balanced meal.

A Peek Inside my Meal Prep World

As I stated earlier on in the book, I am a real person striving and getting real results. Meal prepping works for my lifestyle. I hope this gives you ideas on what and how to eat. Everyone is different so structure your meal plan according to your likes and dislikes. This is an example of what my week looks like and hopefully you can get excited about this adventure as much as I have.

My Day

(These are all approximate times, however I try to stick to them as much as possible)

6:30AM
I prepare a protein shake and a vegetable/fruit mixed drink. However, I may switch up at times and make spinach omelets or oatmeal with fruit.

8AM
Arrive at work and have my breakfast that was prepared earlier.

9AM
I will have a cup of herbal tea with honey and lemon (NO SUGAR).

10:30AM
Snack: Mixed fruit, veggie/fruit drink (prepared previously) or Greek yogurt

12:30 PM

Lunch time: Tilapia, asparagus, sautéed peppers or brown rice

2:30PM

Snack: Fruit, veggies, nuts or Greek yogurt (if I did not have one earlier)

4:30PM

Gym time!!! Prior to the gym I will have fruit or nuts

6PM

Recovery snack/drink (important to have after the gym)
Example: Recovery Drink; Wild Berries, 1 banana, plain Greek yogurt, chia seeds & coconut water

6:30PM

Dinner: Grilled chicken, yams, string beans or mixed greens

I drink lemon water throughout the day
(64+ ounces)

All of the above mentioned meals were all packaged on meal prep day, every Sunday of each week. Can you imagine if I had to get up at 4-5AM to cook these meals? Why do that when I can Meal Prep, grab n go and sleep in a little later each morning.

You will totally benefit from prepping your meals in advance. It contributes to a healthier lifestyle, time and money saver. You win across the board. No more excuses! Get to it! Look and feel good doing it, you can thank me later!

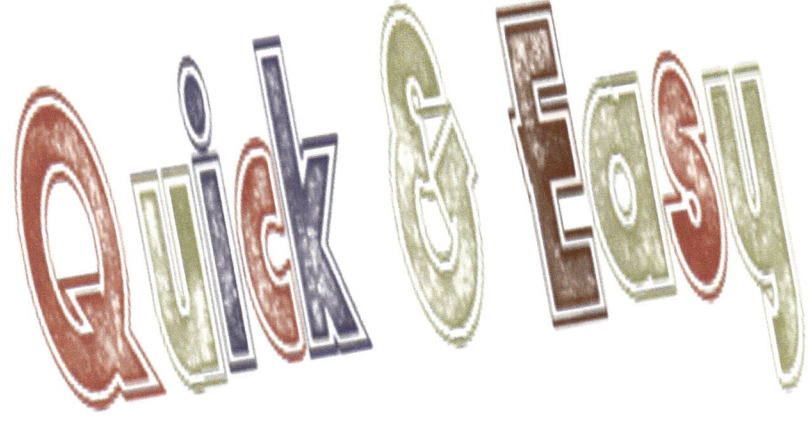

Recipes

There are so many things you can do with chicken breasts, fish and turkey breasts. You can grill, bake and lightly fry (with olive oil). This is one of the reasons I love them. Cooking in large quantities is the best time and money saver. I am by no means a chef. I am someone who is determined to make eating healthy, easy and tasteful. So here are a few of my favorite!

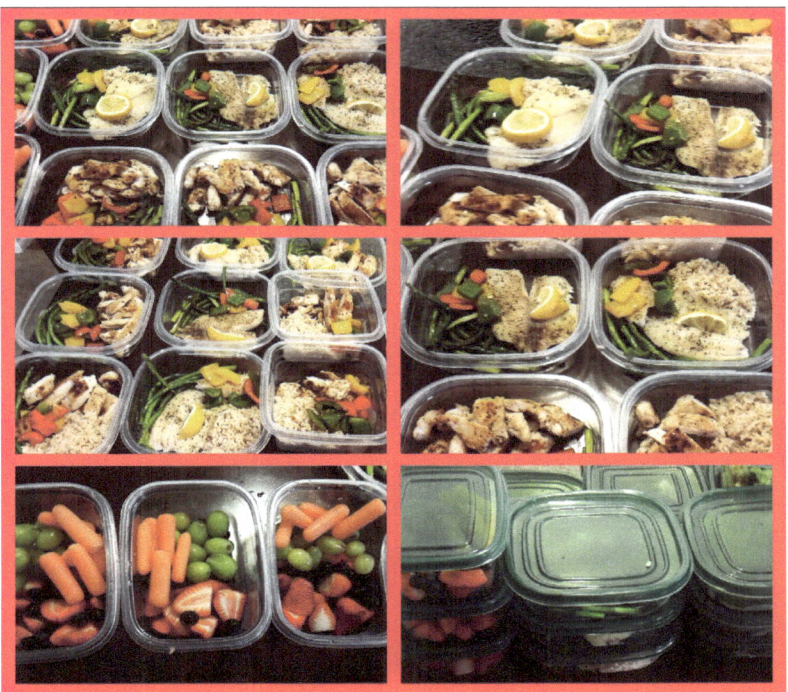

(Pictured above are actual photos of my meal preps)

Recipe #1: Grilled Lemon Chicken Breasts

Ingredients

Extra Virgin Olive Oil
1 lemon
Italian Seasoning blend
1 tbsp. lemon zest
Non-stick cooking spray
1 tsp. ground pepper
Unsalted butter
Lemon wedges

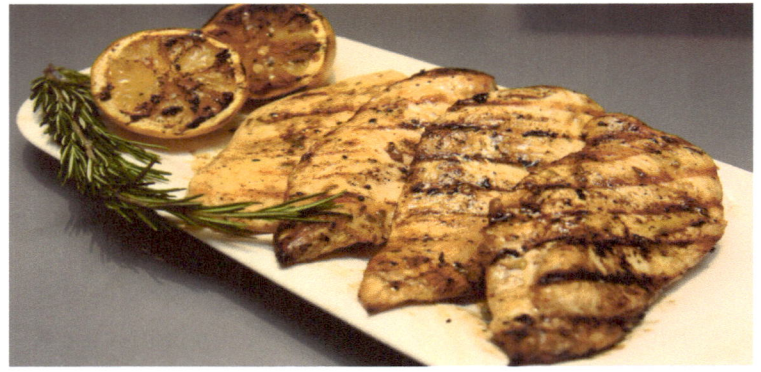

Directions

- Clean and prep chicken breasts (if thick cut slice into as many pieces as possible-$ saver tip)
- Season with Italian seasoning blend or fresh herbs (parsley, oregano, rosemary, thyme, etc.) zest a lemon (mix the lemon zest in with the Italian seasoning) and fresh chopped garlic
- Freshly squeeze the lemon & lightly sprinkle over chicken breast
- Chicken is now ready for the grill (indoor/outdoor)

*Note: You have the option of omitting the lemon juice. The lemon zest will give a great lemon flavor. A whole chicken can also be used for this recipe.

Recipe #2: Stuffed Chicken Breasts

(Sautéed spinach/mozzarella cheese)

Ingredients

Extra Virgin Olive Oil
1 box of frozen or fresh spinach
Italian Seasoning blend
½ tsp. sea salt
1-2 cups of mozzarella cheese
2 cloves of garlic
1 tsp. of red pepper flakes
Unsalted butter

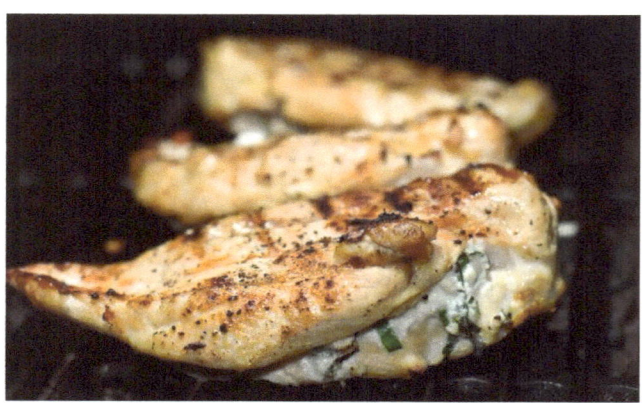

Directions

- Clean and prep chicken breasts
- Season chicken with Italian seasoning/fresh herbs
- To speed up the cooking time you can grill the chicken breasts for couple minutes on each side
- Slice open the chicken breast (create a pocket for the stuffing)
- Sautee spinach in olive oil, garlic and a pinch of sea salt (if you like a kick add red pepper flakes)
- Stuff the chicken breasts with sautéed spinach and small amount of mozzarella cheese (you can also mix the cheese while sautéing the spinach) You also use parmesan cheese
- Place in the 350-375 degree oven and cook for 25-35 minutes (cooking times vary due to oven temps & thickness of chicken breasts)
- Serve with a vegetable & good carb or eat by itself

*You can stuff with any vegetable or food of your choice. Make sure it's a healthy food choice. You can even wrap them in turkey bacon.

Recipe #3: Smothered Chicken Breasts

Ingredients

Extra Virgin Olive Oil
Italian Seasoning blend
2 cans of golden cream of mushroom soup
½ tsp. sea salt
¼ tsp. cayenne pepper
½-cup dry white wine
Unsalted butter
Lemon wedges when serving

Directions

- Clean and prep chicken breasts
- Season chicken breasts with fresh herbs or Italian blend
- Grill the chicken breasts or cook half way through in a 350-375 degree oven
- Place in a baking pan and add a low-sodium *golden* cream of mushroom soup or you can make your own
- Continue cooking in the oven (you can add more soup if needed while cooking)
- Serve hot with veggies and good carb of your choice

Recipe #4: Baked Tilapia

Ingredients

Extra Virgin Olive Oil
2-3 cloves of garlic
Italian Seasoning blend
½ tsp. sea salt
1 tsp. of parsley
1 lemon
Bell peppers (multi-color)
Unsalted butter
Lemon wedges

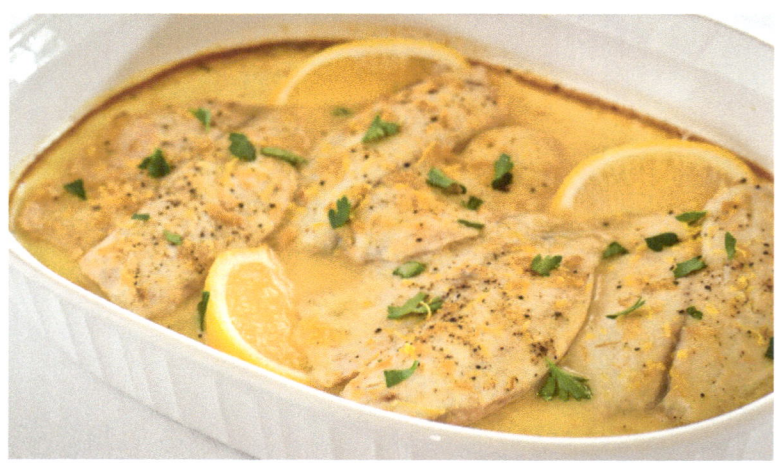

Directions

- Prepare the tilapia (fish of your choice)
- Place in a pan season with Italian seasoning or fresh herbs (you can also individually wrap each piece in foil)
- Place some unsalted butter in the pan (you can melt about a tablespoon or so depending on the amount of fish) in a pot, chop fresh garlic and mix with butter once you remove pot from stove and pour over the fish
- Squeeze lemon juice over the fish and cut lemon slices and put on top of each piece
- Slice some peppers (multi-color) and place on each piece (option of using onions)
- Place in oven at 350 degrees; I haven't given a specific cooking time; it will vary depending on the amount and thickness of the pieces. You do not want to dry out the fish, so keep checking on it. I wouldn't cook for more than 25 minutes.
- When done you can garnish with parsley

Recipe #5: Pepper Cups (Stuffed Peppers)

Ingredients

Extra Virgin Olive Oil
Bell peppers
1lb of ground turkey
2-3 cloves of garlic
1 tomato
½ tsp. sea salt
1 cup mozzarella cheese
Beans and olives optional

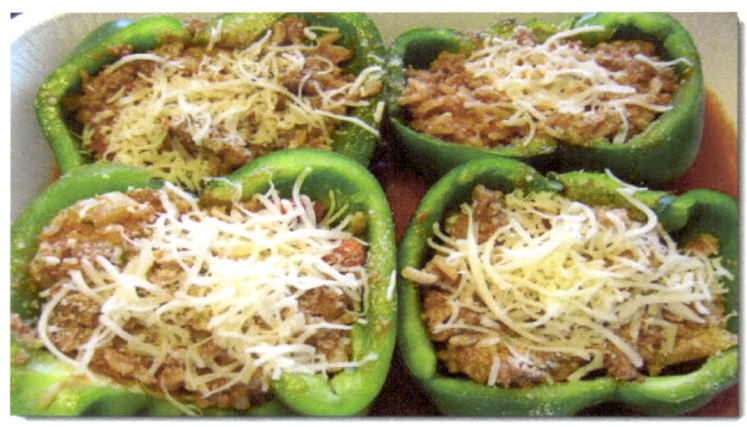

Directions

- Most cut the tops off, but I cut them in half. It makes them more manageable when eating (use tri-color peppers makes it different)
- Coat them with a little olive oil & place them on a baking sheet
- Place in the over at 350°F for a few minutes
- Brown some ground turkey with onions, fresh garlic, diced tomato and Italian Seasoning blend or fresh herbs (optional) & sea salt you can also use tomato sauce, up to you
- Scoop the cooked ground turkey into each bell pepper and place back in the oven. Top with cheese (not too much)
- Optional: Mix beans & black olives in the ground turkey
- Serve hot with brown rice or other good carb & veggies

Have fun with this recipe! You can stuff them with anything!
Vegan alternative: Use quinoa & black beans for stuffing

Recipe #6: Honey Glazed Salmon

Ingredients

Extra Virgin Olive Oil
Italian Seasoning blend
¼ cup honey
1 tsp. Worcestershire sauce
1 tbsp. Dijon mustard
Unsalted butter

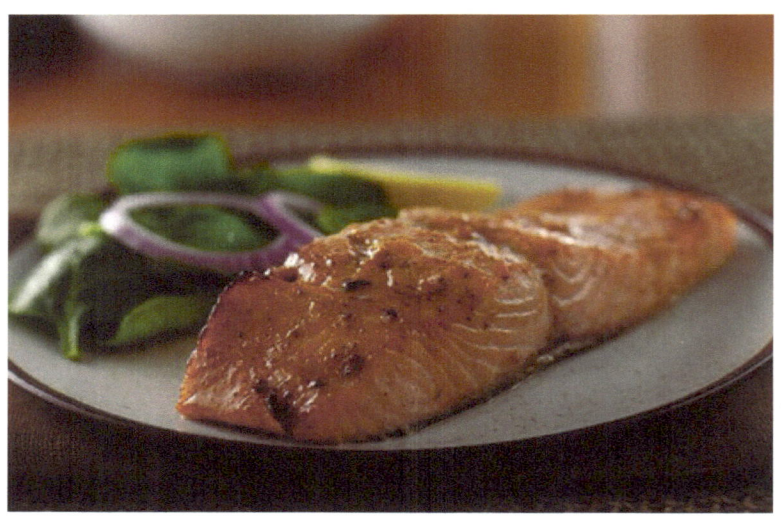

Directions

- Slice salmon into 2 inch strips ($ saver)
- Rub each piece with a little olive oil
- Season with Italian seasoning blend
- Line pan with foil
- Place a 400°F oven for 10-15 minutes (cooking times vary due to thickness of pieces)
- Prepare the glaze: ¼ cup honey, 1tsp Worcestershire sauce, 1-2 tbsp. of Dijon mustard, 1tbsp melted unsalted butter
- Remove salmon from oven, pour on the glaze
- Place back in oven for another 5 minutes or so (do not overcook)

Recipe #7: Spicy Garlic Shrimp

Ingredients

Extra Virgin Olive Oil
2-3 cloves of garlic
1 tsp. ground cumin
½ tsp. sea salt
¼ tsp. cayenne pepper
½-1 cup dry white wine
1 pound peeled/deveined raw shrimp
1 tbsp. fresh lemon juice
1 tbsp. unsalted butter

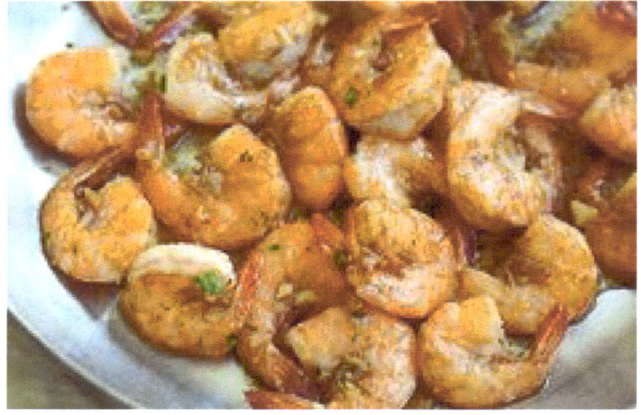

Directions

- Heat olive oil in a skillet
- Add cumin, garlic, sea salt, cayenne pepper, 1 tbsp. of unsalted butter & stir for approximately 20-30 seconds
- Stir in dry white cooking wine and bring to a simmer
- Add in shrimp and cook until pink about 3 minutes
- Remove skillet from heat and add lemon juice
- Garnish with parsley or cilantro and serve over 100% whole wheat pasta, brown rice, quinoa, vegetable such as asparagus

***Cooking times may vary due to amount & size of shrimp.

Desserts

Oh yes, we have to have desserts! I have a sweet tooth and I had to find a way to tame it. You can still enjoy certain things with some alterations. When you deprive yourself you end up over indulging and making bad choices.
So here we go!

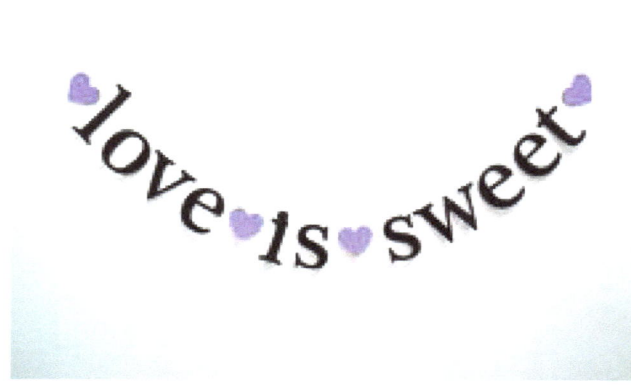

Recipe #7: Homemade Popsicles

- You need Popsicle molds-I pre-freeze them before I place the mixture in. It speeds up the freezing process!
- Prepare fresh fruits of your liking or that are in season (Use a wide variety of fresh fruits, pineapples, apples, blueberries, mango, oranges, strawberries, berries, watermelon, banana, etc.)
- Place in a blender, smoothie maker whatever you have and pour in a low sugar-all natural juice (orange, apple, etc.) or almond milk
- Blend until thin consistency (juice); Optional: Place chunks of fruit in the molds prior to pouring in juice mixture
- Pour mixture in Popsicle molds and place in freezer
- Doesn't get any easier than that! Great for summer and those spare of the moment cravings!

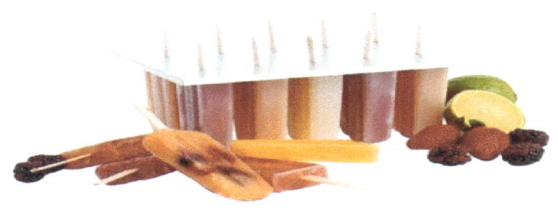

Recipe #6: Parfaits

Ingredients

**1-2 cups Plain, Vanilla or Lemon Greek
yogurt**
Fruits of your choice
**¼-half cup Organic Granola or Graham
cracker crumbs**
1 tsp. Honey

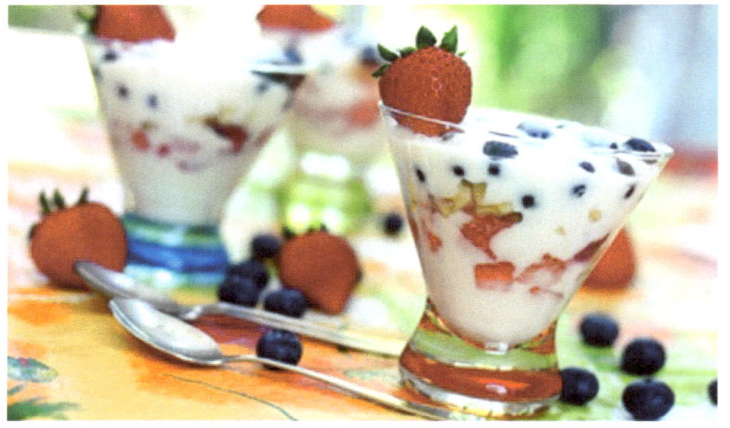

Directions

- Mix honey into Greek yogurt to sweeten
- Place a layer of either granola or Greek yogurt in a cup to start
- Continue alternating layers in the cup of Greek yogurt, granola and fruit (make as many layers as you like)
- Garnish with a little granola or graham cracker crumbs
- ENJOY

How simply is this to make? Make a few cups so you can grab one when you need something sweet. Great tasting and great for you!

Snack Ideas

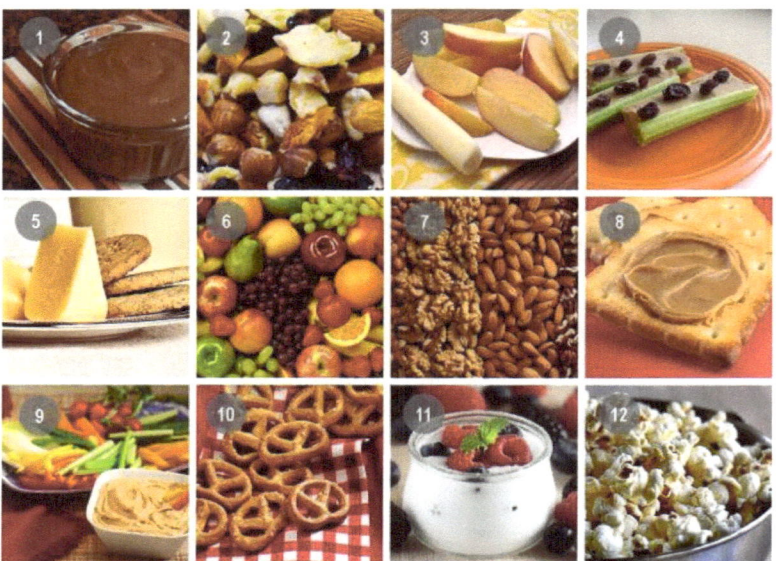

(Photo courtesy of Live Well @ UMD)

1. 1/2 cup low-fat pudding
2. 1/4 cup reduced-fat trail mix
3. 1 reduced fat string cheese & 1 medium apple
4. 2 celery stalks with 2 tbsp. peanut butter and 2 tbsp. raisins
5. 1 oz. low-fat cheese and 3-5 whole wheat crackers
6. 1 medium fruit or 1/2 cup fruit in its own juice
7. 1 oz. mixed nuts
8. 3 whole wheat crackers with peanut butter & 6 oz. skim milk
9. 1 cup raw veggies with 2 tbsp. reduced-fat dressing or 1/4 cup hummus
10. 1 oz. whole wheat pretzels, lightly salted
11. 8 oz. non-fat yogurt with 1/2 cup berries
12. 3 cup air-popped popcorn

Here are a few suggestions for snacks. I know I can't be the only one that has cravings.

- Jell-O (no sugar added) Make your own and add fruits to it. Top it off with a little whipped cream!
- Pretzels (Unsalted) I actually have mine with a little mustard
- Fruit salads are the best. When you make your own you can put the fruits you enjoy. You can even throw some honey in with it!
- Frozen yogurt- not from the store! Buy some plain Greek yogurt. Put some honey & fruits and place in the freezer. You literally will have frozen yogurt!
- Frozen blueberries- I freeze blueberries so while watching a movie I can eat them like popcorn! Try it!
- Popcorn – Sorry no butter! You can lightly sprinkle some sea salt and garlic on the popcorn (while it's hot) and you will love the taste. Sometimes I also sprinkle cinnamon on the popcorn & a little brown sugar
- Grilled pineapples
- Baked apples with cinnamon and nutmeg or applesauce
  There are tons of snacks you can enjoy!

Bon Appétit

Danielle's Protein Shake Recipes

Here are some of my favorites…Enjoy!

Lemon Berry Delight

- 3-4 ice cubes
- 10-12 oz. of almond milk (or water)
- 1 tsp. of lemon juice (fresh squeezed)
- 8-10 blueberries or wild berries
- 1 scoop of vanilla protein powder

Banana Almond

- 3-4 ice cubes
- 10-12 oz. of almond milk (or water)
- 1 banana
- 1 tsp. of almond extract
- 1 scoop of vanilla or chocolate protein powder

Berry Berrilicious

- 3-4 ice cubes
- 10-12 oz. of almond milk (or water)
- 3-4 strawberries
- 8-10 blueberries
- 1 scoop of protein powder

Peachy Cream

- 3-4 ice cubes
- 10-12 oz. of almond milk (or water)
- Add fresh or frozen peaches (4-5)

- 1 scoop of vanilla protein powder

Cinnamon Apple Turnover
- 3-4 ice cubes
- 10-12 oz. of almond milk (or water)
- Add 1 tsp. of cinnamon
- ½ green apple (sliced)
- 1 scoop of vanilla protein powder

Cocoa Fever
- 3-4 ice cubes
- 10-12 oz. of almond milk (or water)
- 1 tsp. of pure cocoa powder
- 1 scoop of either vanilla or chocolate protein powder

Coconut Cream
- 3-4 ice cubes
- 10-12 oz. of almond milk (or water)
- 2 tsp. of shredded coconut
- 1 scoop of vanilla protein powder

*Use 1-2 scoops of Protein Powder; depends on your goals

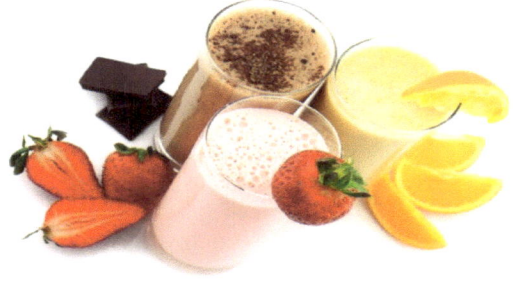

FOOD JOURNAL SECTION

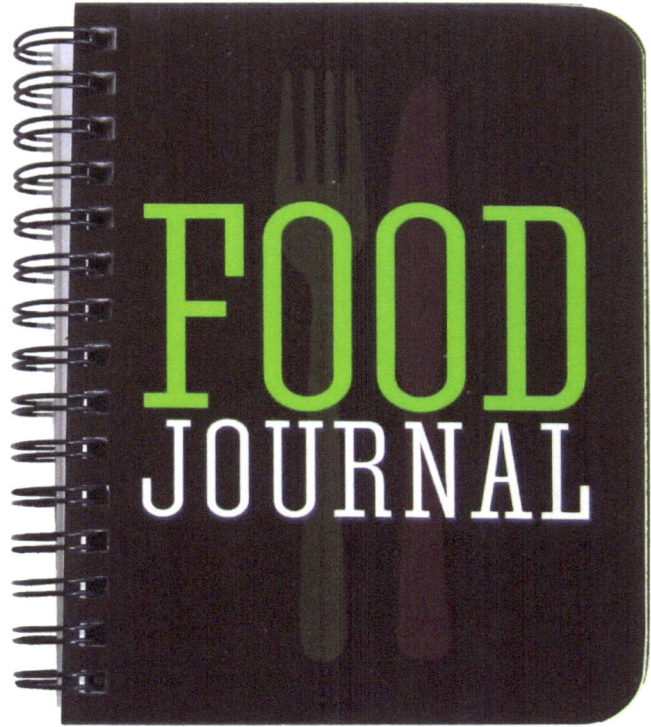

I have supplied you with a food journal that will help you keep track of your journey. I suggest making copies before you start using it. Even if you do it for the first week or two of this new meal prep journey, it will help you stay focused and make necessary adjustments! You should also keep track of your emotions daily. It will help you discover if you are an emotional eater as well as identify the stressors in your life. We must be healthy in our mind, body and spirit! You're the only one that has control over all three!

```
┌─────────────────────────────────────────────────────────┐
│                  Weekly Food Journal                      │
│        Journal Day #_____        Date:_____          │
└─────────────────────────────────────────────────────────┘
```

Lemon water: ____Y/____N

Water (at least eight glasses): □ □ □ □ □ □ □ □

Other beverages:

Supplements: ____Y/____N

Breakfast: _____

_____

Mid-morning snack: _____

_____

Lunch: _____

_____

Mid-afternoon snack: _____

_____

Dinner: _____

_____

Evening Snack: _____

_____

Exercise:

_____

How I felt today:
(Obstacles, milestones, emotional changes, stressors)

_____
_____
_____
_____
_____
_____
_____
_____
_____
_____
_____
_____
_____
_____
_____
_____
_____
_____
_____
_____
_____
_____
_____
_____
_____
_____
_____
_____

30-DAY SEXY BEAST CHALLENGE
Sorry Fellas…this group is for women only! ☺

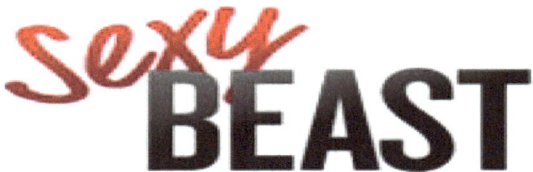

      If you would like support with your healthy lifestyle change, look us up on Facebook. We've had 6 (30 day) cycles in this group and there's been much success! Women have lost a tremendous amount of weight and inches. It's a support group and we found with accountability people are more sustainable to change. To participate you must set goals, post photos of your daily meal intakes/workouts and encourage each other. We are a community that inspires, shares stories of our success and our struggles. We also share recipes, exercise routines and track our progress.

Support is one of the 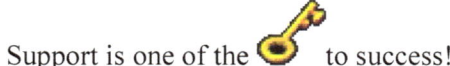 to success!

Please look us up on Facebook or email us @ sexybeastchallenge@gmail.com for more information.

Look & Act like a lady but train like a Beast!

The Author
Danielle Richardson
© 2015

Diary of a Fit MOMMY!

www.ingramcontent.com/pod-product-compliance
Lightning Source LLC
Chambersburg PA
CBHW041514280526
45792CB00004B/1254